WALL PILATES FOR SENIORS OVER THE AGE OF 60

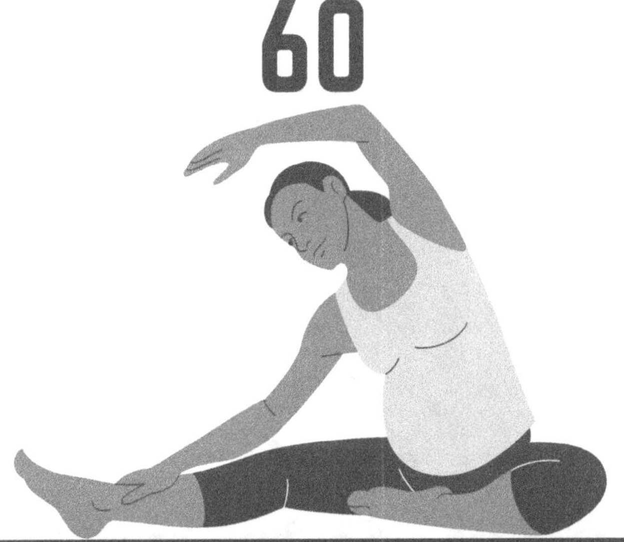

Improve Strength, Flexibility and Balance Using Low-Impact Pilates, The Complete Guide to Home Wall Workouts for Adults Over 60 to Enhance Mobility

Troy Vhodes

Copyright © 2024 by Troy Vhodes

Table of Contents

Advanced Wall Pilates Techniques:
   - Progressing Your Routine for Ongoing Improvement
   - Challenging Yourself Safely

Conclusion

Introduction

In the realm of fitness, where strength meets grace, and age is no barrier to transformation, there exists a pathway to vibrant well-being that transcends the ordinary. Welcome to "Wall Pilates for Seniors Over 60" – a holistic guide crafted to ignite the flame of vitality within you.

Picture this:
In the quiet moments of your day, envision yourself standing tall, embodying a strength you never thought possible. Picture the graceful flow of movements, each one enhancing your flexibility and balance. Imagine the serene confidence that comes from a body in harmony, a body that has discovered the power of low-impact Pilates against the sturdy backdrop of your own home wall.

But this journey is more than just exercises; it's a transformation:
Transform your Strength, Flexibility, and Balance, these aren't just words; they are the promises whispered by each Pilates move. The Complete Guide within these pages unveils the secrets to unlocking your body's potential. Imagine rediscovering the strength of your youth, the flexibility of your prime, and the balance that keeps you moving forward.

Embrace Mobility, Stability, and Posture, the pillars of graceful aging. Our guide is your companion on this quest for not just physical well-being but a holistic elevation of your entire being. Through low-impact Pilates, discover a renewed sense of mobility, a steadfast stability, and a posture that radiates confidence.

Did you know:
Each page is filled with the wisdom and passion that fueled my own transformative journey with Wall Pilates. Here, you're not just reading a guide; you're stepping into a world where fitness becomes a celebration, and every movement is a step towards a healthier, happier you.

As a famous saying goes:
Strength does not come from the body. It comes from the will." - A mantra embraced by athletes, trainers, and now, by you as you embark on this transformative journey.

Embark on a journey with me:
Imagine the joy of conquering fitness challenges you once thought insurmountable. Consider the fulfillment of reclaiming the vitality that time may have subtly taken away. "Wall Pilates for Seniors Over 60" is not just a guide; it's an invitation to a transformative experience that awaits you on the other side of these pages.

Are you ready to redefine your fitness story?
Turn the page and step into a world where strength, flexibility, and balance converge to sculpt a healthier, more vibrant version of you. The first chapter beckons – let's embark on this empowering journey together. Your transformation begins now.

Chapter 1
The Foundation of Wall Pilates
Exploring Low-Impact Exercises

As you step into the realm of Wall Pilates, consider this chapter as the rhythmic pulse that sets the tone for your journey. We're not just delving into exercises; we're exploring the very heartbeat of transformative fitness. So, let's dive in, shall we?

Let's Talk Low-Impact: A Kind Approach to Strength

In the world of fitness, "low-impact" isn't just a term; it's a philosophy. Imagine the gentle cadence of movements that embrace your body, whispering promises of strength without strain. Picture a workout where each motion is a graceful dance with your own capabilities, an exploration of what your body can achieve without the jarring impact.

What Makes Pilates Low-Impact?

Let's demystify the magic. Pilates, at its essence, is a symphony of controlled movements, choreographed to sculpt your physique without subjecting it to the stress of high-impact exercises. It's like crafting a masterpiece with finesse, each stroke purposeful, every note deliberate.

Consider the analogy of a dancer on a stage. They glide, they leap, they twirl – yet, there's a softness, an elegance that defines their every move. Pilates echoes this ethos. It's a dance with resistance, a conversation between your body and the wall, where impact takes a back seat, and the art of motion reigns supreme.

The Harmony of Controlled Energy

In Wall Pilates, low-impact isn't a compromise; it's a revelation. It's about channeling energy with precision, about sculpting your strength with a gentleness that invites sustainability. As you explore each exercise, feel the harmony between muscle engagement and controlled energy – a delicate balance that transforms workouts into a journey of self-discovery.

Why Low-Impact Matters for Seniors Over 60

This isn't just about exercise; it's about crafting an experience tailored to your unique needs. For seniors over 60, low-impact Pilates becomes the compass guiding you towards a fitter, more agile future. It's a celebration of your body's resilience, a testament to the fact that fitness is not just for the young – it's for those who choose vitality at every age.

So, as you embark on this exploration of low-impact Pilates, envision each movement as a brushstroke on the canvas of your well-being. The foundation is set, and the journey has just begun. Join me as we navigate the artistry of Wall Pilates and discover the transformative power of controlled, low-impact exercises. Let the rhythm of your fitness journey resonate with the gentle beat of Wall Pilates.

Why It's Ideal for Seniors Over 60: A Symphony of Benefits

Entering the golden years is not a signal to slow down; it's an invitation to discover new avenues of well-being. In the realm of fitness, especially for those aged 60 and beyond, Wall Pilates stands as a beacon of idealism, offering a unique blend of benefits that resonate harmoniously with the needs of seniors. Let's unravel why Wall Pilates is not just an exercise routine but a tailored symphony of wellness for this vibrant demographic.

1. Gentle on Joints, Mighty on Results:

Wall Pilates embraces a philosophy of low-impact, a quality that becomes increasingly crucial as we age. For seniors over 60, the gentleness of these exercises becomes a boon for joints that have weathered decades of movement. Unlike high-impact workouts that may strain or stress joints, Pilates on the wall provides a nurturing environment where strength is built without unnecessary wear and tear. It's the gentle giant of fitness, preserving joint health while sculpting strength.

2. Customizable for Every Fitness Level:

One size does not fit all, especially when it comes to fitness for seniors. Wall Pilates acknowledges this diversity and offers a customizable approach. Whether you're a fitness enthusiast or just starting your wellness journey, each exercise can be adapted to your unique fitness level. This adaptability ensures that seniors of varying physical conditions can engage in a workout that suits their needs, promoting inclusivity in the pursuit of fitness.

3. Enhances Core Strength and Stability:

Core strength is the backbone of physical well-being, especially for seniors who may face challenges related to balance and stability. Wall Pilates, with its emphasis on controlled movements and engagement of the core, becomes a powerful ally in fortifying this vital area. As we age, maintaining a strong core is not just about aesthetics but a key factor in preventing falls and supporting overall stability.

4. Fosters Mind-Body Connection:

Beyond the physical, Wall Pilates invites seniors to cultivate a profound mind-body connection. The deliberate, controlled movements demand focus and mindfulness, turning each session into a therapeutic experience. For seniors navigating the complexities of aging, this mental engagement becomes a sanctuary, offering not just physical exercise but a holistic escape into self-awareness and mental well-being.

5. Promotes Flexibility and Mobility:

Flexibility is the elixir of youthful movement, and Wall Pilates infuses each routine with the promise of enhanced flexibility. The wall becomes a support, enabling seniors to explore a range of motions that contribute to improved flexibility and mobility. These exercises, designed to flow seamlessly from one to another, foster a sense of fluidity in movement, a quality that becomes increasingly valuable as we age.

6. Tailored for Home Comfort:

Recognizing the unique needs of seniors, Wall Pilates brings the gym to your home. The routines are crafted with the understanding that accessibility and comfort are paramount. No need for intimidating gym equipment or rigorous commutes. Your home becomes the sanctuary where you embark on a journey of rejuvenation, blending the convenience of home workouts with the effectiveness of Pilates.

In essence, Wall Pilates for Seniors Over 60 is not merely a fitness routine; it's a tailored symphony of benefits that celebrates the wisdom, strength, and vibrancy of this age group. It's an invitation to move, to explore, and to redefine what it means to age gracefully. Join the movement, and let the wall be your canvas for a masterpiece of well-being.

Setting Up Your Home Wall Workout Space

In the realm of Wall Pilates, your home transforms into more than just a living space; it becomes a sanctuary for your fitness journey. Setting up your home wall workout space is not merely a practical task – it's an intentional act of creating an environment where wellness thrives. Let's embark on this journey of crafting a haven, considering both safety and comfort, along with the essential equipment and accessories that will elevate your Wall Pilates experience.

1. Creating a Safe and Comfortable Environment:

a. Choose the Right Space:

Select a space with enough room to move freely. Ensure it is well-lit and ventilated, creating an inviting ambiance. A dedicated corner of a room or even a cleared-out area in the living room can serve as your fitness haven.

b. Secure Flooring:

Invest in a non-slip mat or carpet to provide a stable surface. This not only enhances safety during exercises but also adds a touch of comfort to your routines. Your feet should feel grounded and secure, fostering confidence in every movement.

c. Remove Obstacles:

Clear the space of any potential hazards. Keep furniture, cords, or any other obstacles out of the workout area. A clutter-free space not only ensures safety but also allows you to move seamlessly through your Pilates routine.

d. *Adequate Lighting:*

Illumination matters. Ensure that the space is well-lit to enhance visibility and create a positive atmosphere. Natural light is ideal, but if that's not possible, consider investing in good quality, adjustable lighting.

2. Essential Equipment and Accessories:

a. *Wall Anchor or Mount:*

The wall is your anchor in Wall Pilates. Ensure it's sturdy and capable of supporting your body weight. If you don't have a suitable wall, consider wall mounts or anchors designed for fitness purposes.

b. *Exercise Mat:*

A comfortable, non-slip exercise mat is essential for floor exercises. It provides cushioning and support, enhancing your comfort during the routines.

c. *Resistance Bands:*

These versatile accessories add an extra layer of challenge to your exercises. From aiding in stretches to providing resistance during movements, resistance bands are a valuable addition to your Pilates toolkit.

d. *Stability Ball:*

For exercises that engage your core and balance, a stability ball is a fantastic addition. It adds variety to your routines and helps improve stability.

e. Pilates Ring:

This small but mighty tool is excellent for targeting specific muscle groups. It adds resistance and diversity to your exercises, enhancing the overall effectiveness of your Pilates workout.

f. Water and Towel:

Stay hydrated throughout your workout, and keep a towel handy. Hydration is key to a successful fitness session, and a towel ensures you stay comfortable, especially if you're breaking a sweat.

In crafting your home wall workout space, remember that it's more than a physical setting – it's a personal haven for your wellness journey. By paying attention to safety, comfort, and the essential equipment, you're not just creating a space to exercise; you're creating a retreat for self-care and transformation. Let this space be a reflection of your commitment to well-being, and let the wall be the canvas for your journey to strength, flexibility, and balance.

Chapter 2
Getting Started with Wall Pilates
Basic Wall Pilates Poses

Welcome to the gateway of your Wall Pilates journey! In this chapter, we'll navigate the basics, laying the foundation for the transformative path that lies ahead. Let's dive into the world of Wall Pilates poses, starting with the gentle stretches and warm-ups that will awaken your body and prepare it for the graceful movements to come.

In the canvas of Wall Pilates, each pose is a brushstroke, contributing to the masterpiece of your fitness. Let's explore these fundamental poses that form the core of your practice, infusing strength, flexibility, and balance into every fiber of your being.

a. The Wall Lean:

- Stand facing the wall with feet hip-width apart.
- Gently press your palms against the wall at shoulder height.
- Lean your body forward, maintaining a straight line from head to heels.
- Feel the stretch in your chest, shoulders, and upper back.
- Hold for 15-30 seconds, breathing deeply.

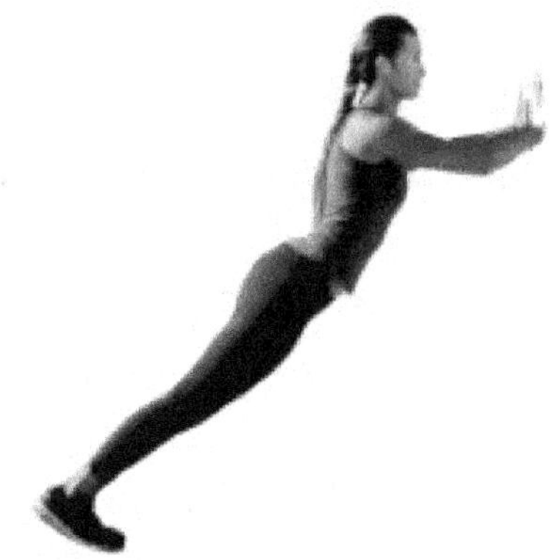

- Position yourself with your back against the wall and feet shoulder-width apart.
- Lower your body into a seated position, as if sitting in an imaginary chair.
- Ensure your knees are directly above your ankles.
- Hold for 15-30 seconds, engaging your thighs and glutes.
- Rise slowly, maintaining control.

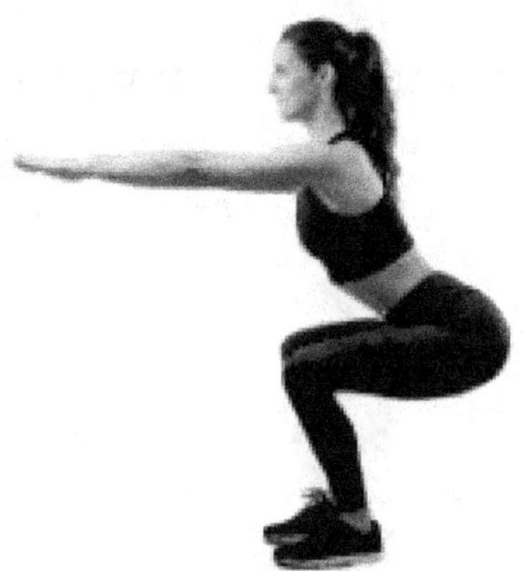

c. Wall Plank:

- Face the wall and place your hands on it at shoulder height.
- Step back until your body is in a straight line from head to heels.
- Engage your core and hold the position for 20-40 seconds.
- Focus on maintaining a neutral spine and steady breathing.

d. Wall Bridge:

- Lie on your back with feet flat against the wall and knees bent.
- Press your lower back into the floor, engaging your core.
- Lift your hips toward the ceiling, creating a straight line from shoulders to knees.
- Hold for 15-30 seconds, feeling the activation in your glutes and hamstrings.
- Lower your hips back down with control.

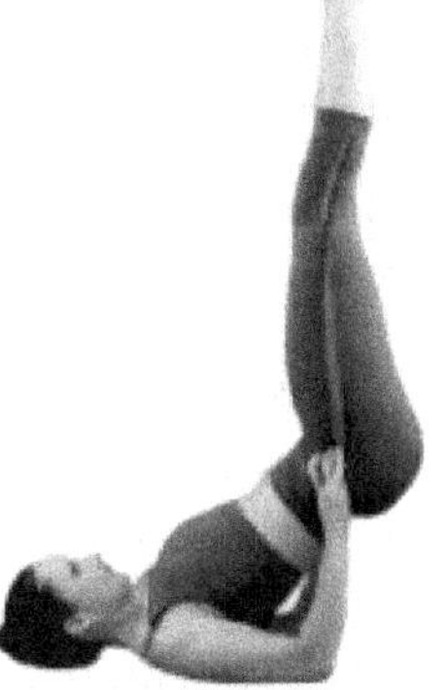

Gentle Stretches and Warm-ups: Preparing the Canvas

Before immersing yourself in the poses, let's lay the groundwork with gentle stretches and warm-ups. These movements not only increase blood flow but also improve flexibility, making each pose more accessible and effective.

a. Neck Stretch:

- Slowly tilt your head to one side, bringing your ear toward your shoulder.
- Hold for 15 seconds, feeling the stretch along the side of your neck.
- Repeat on the other side.

b. Shoulder Rolls:

- Lift your shoulders up toward your ears, then roll them back in a circular motion.
- Perform 10 backward rolls, then reverse direction for 10 forward rolls.

c. Arm Circles:

- Extend your arms to the sides at shoulder height.
- Make small circles in a clockwise motion for 20 seconds, then switch to counterclockwise.

d. Leg Swings:

- Stand facing the wall, using it for support.
- Swing one leg forward and backward in a controlled motion.
- Repeat for 10 swings on each leg.

- Lift one foot off the ground and rotate your ankle in a circular motion.
- Perform 10 circles in each direction, then switch to the other ankle.

As you embark on these basic Wall Pilates poses and gentle warm-ups, remember that this chapter is your initiation into a journey of mindful movement. Each pose and stretch contributes to the symphony of your wellness, fostering strength, flexibility, and balance. So, let the canvas of your practice unfold, and let each movement be a stroke of self-care and transformation. The wall is your support, and the poses are your expressions of strength and grace. Welcome to the artistry of Wall Pilates.

Breathing Techniques for Relaxation: Inhale Serenity, Exhale Tension

As you delve into the tranquil world of Wall Pilates, the rhythm of your breath becomes a guiding force, weaving through each movement and creating a symphony of relaxation. In this chapter, we explore the art of mindful breathing techniques – an essential aspect of your practice that not only enhances your physical performance but also serves as a gateway to inner calmness and serenity.

Understanding the Power of Breath:
Before we embark on specific techniques, let's recognize the profound influence that conscious breathing can have on our well-being. The breath is a bridge between the conscious and subconscious, a tool that can be harnessed to calm the mind, reduce stress, and enhance overall relaxation. In Wall Pilates, aligning your breath with movement becomes a cornerstone of the practice, allowing you to move with intention and grace.

a. Diaphragmatic Breathing:
- Sit or lie down comfortably, placing one hand on your chest and the other on your abdomen.
- Inhale deeply through your nose, allowing your abdomen to expand as you fill your lungs with air.
- Exhale slowly through pursed lips, feeling your abdomen contract.
- Repeat for 5-10 breaths, focusing on the rise and fall of your abdomen.

b. 4-7-8 Technique:

- Inhale quietly through your nose for a count of 4.
- Hold your breath for a count of 7.
- Exhale completely through your mouth for a count of 8.
- Repeat this cycle for 4 breaths, gradually increasing as you become more comfortable.

c. Box Breathing:

- Inhale slowly through your nose for a count of 4.
- Hold your breath for a count of 4.
- Exhale completely through your mouth for a count of 4.
- Pause for a count of 4 before inhaling again.
- Repeat this cycle for several breaths, allowing a sense of calm to envelop you.

d. Alternate Nostril Breathing (Nadi Shodhana):

- Sit comfortably, using your right thumb to close off your right nostril.
- Inhale deeply through your left nostril.
- Close your left nostril with your right ring finger, releasing your right nostril.
- Exhale completely through your right nostril.
- Inhale through your right nostril, then close it off and exhale through your left nostril.
- Repeat this cycle for 5-10 rounds, focusing on the gentle flow of breath.

Integrating Breath into Wall Pilates:

As you perform Wall Pilates poses, synchronize your breath with movement. Inhale during the preparatory phase, and exhale as you engage in the movement. Allow your breath to be a continuous flow, guiding each pose with a sense of ease and presence. The intentional pairing of breath and movement not only enhances the effectiveness of the exercises but also creates a meditative quality to your practice.

In the tapestry of Wall Pilates, these breathing techniques serve as threads of relaxation, weaving through each pose and creating a seamless connection between body and mind. Embrace the power of your breath, allowing it to be a source of tranquility as you embark on this journey of physical and mental well-being. Inhale serenity, exhale tension – welcome to the harmonious dance of breath and movement in Wall Pilates.

Understanding Your Body's Needs

In the exploration of Wall Pilates, recognizing and responding to the unique needs of your body is paramount. This chapter delves into the intricacies of understanding your body's requirements, emphasizing the importance of tailoring Wall Pilates workouts to accommodate different fitness levels. It's not just about the exercises; it's about creating an inclusive space where every participant, regardless of their fitness background, can embark on a journey of well-being.

Body Awareness: The First Step to Tailoring Workouts
Before delving into the specifics of tailoring workouts, let's underscore the significance of body awareness. Understanding your body's cues, limitations, and strengths is the compass that guides your Wall Pilates practice. Take a moment to connect with your body, listening attentively to its signals during each movement. This mindfulness lays the foundation for an adaptive and personalized fitness experience.

Tailoring Workouts for Different Fitness Levels: A Multifaceted Approach

a. Beginners: Establishing Foundations

Introduction to Basic Poses:
- Start with foundational poses, gradually introducing the primary Wall Pilates moves.
- Focus on proper form and alignment, ensuring a solid understanding of the basics.

Modified Movements:
- Offer simplified versions of exercises to build confidence.
- Utilize props like cushions or resistance bands for added support.

Shorter Sessions:
- Begin with shorter sessions and progressively extend the duration as fitness improves.
- Emphasize quality over quantity to prevent fatigue or strain.

b. Intermediate: Building on Foundations

Variations and Progressions:
- Introduce variations to basic poses, challenging participants to deepen their practice.
- Progress to more advanced moves as strength and flexibility develop.

Increased Repetitions:
- Gradually increase the number of repetitions, promoting endurance.
- Encourage participants to explore controlled movements with a focus on breath.

Integration of Props:
- Incorporate additional props like stability balls or Pilates rings to add variety.
- Tailor sessions to specific goals, such as core strength or improved flexibility.

c. Advanced: Elevating the Practice

Complex Sequences:
- Introduce complex sequences that demand a higher level of coordination.
- Encourage fluid transitions between poses, fostering a seamless flow.

Targeted Muscle Engagement:
- Emphasize precise muscle engagement for an advanced level of sculpting.
- Incorporate isometric holds and dynamic movements for a comprehensive workout.

Personalized Challenges:
- Tailor challenges based on individual goals and preferences.
- Provide options for participants to choose their preferred level of difficulty.

Key Principles for Tailoring:

a. Flexibility in Programming:
- Design sessions with flexibility, allowing participants to choose exercises that suit their comfort level.
- Provide options for modifications and advancements, catering to individual preferences.

b. Individualized Guidance:
- Offer personalized guidance during sessions, addressing specific concerns or modifications.
- Encourage open communication to understand participants' needs and adapt accordingly.

- Incorporate progress checks to track improvements.
- Adjust workouts based on individual progress, ensuring a gradual and sustainable development.

In essence, understanding your body's needs and tailoring Wall Pilates workouts for different fitness levels transforms each session into a personalized journey. It's an inclusive approach that honors the diverse needs of participants, fostering a sense of empowerment and accomplishment. As you engage in Wall Pilates, let this understanding be your compass, guiding you toward a wellness experience that is as unique as you are. Tailor your practice, embrace the journey, and revel in the transformative power of Wall Pilates at every fitness level

Addressing Common Concerns and Health Conditions: Navigating Wellness with Wall Pilates

Embarking on a fitness journey, especially one as nuanced as Wall Pilates, requires a mindful consideration of individual health concerns and conditions. This chapter serves as a guide, addressing common concerns and providing insights on how to adapt Wall Pilates to accommodate various health scenarios.

Before You Begin: Consultation and Communication
Prior to engaging in any exercise routine, including Wall Pilates, it is advisable to consult with a healthcare professional, especially if you have existing health conditions or concerns. Open communication with your healthcare provider ensures a safe and tailored approach to your fitness journey.

Common Concerns and Adaptations:

a. Back Pain:
Concern:
Individuals experiencing back pain may worry about exacerbating their condition through exercise.

Adaptations:
- Focus on gentle movements that engage the core without straining the back.
- Modify poses, choosing those that provide support and minimize stress on the spine.
- Gradually introduce exercises, paying attention to comfort and avoiding any movements that cause discomfort.

b. Joint Issues (Arthritis, Osteoarthritis):

Concern:

Joint pain or stiffness can be a significant concern for individuals with arthritis or osteoarthritis.

Adaptations:
- Opt for low-impact exercises that promote joint mobility without excessive stress.
- Incorporate controlled movements, avoiding sudden or jarring actions.
- Utilize props or modifications to reduce strain on affected joints.

c. Cardiovascular Conditions:

Concern:

Individuals with cardiovascular conditions may be cautious about engaging in activities that elevate heart rate.

Adaptations:
- Emphasize controlled breathing techniques to promote relaxation and maintain steady heart rate.
- Begin with shorter sessions and gradually increase intensity based on individual tolerance.
- Encourage regular breaks and hydration during workouts.

Concern:

Those with balance concerns may worry about the stability required for certain exercises.

Adaptations:
- Incorporate exercises near a supportive surface, such as a wall or sturdy chair, to enhance stability.
- Emphasize poses that improve balance gradually, with an emphasis on safety.

e. Pregnancy:

Concern:

Pregnant individuals may be uncertain about the suitability of certain movements.

Adaptations:
- Avoid exercises that involve lying flat on the back after the first trimester.
- Modify poses to accommodate the changing center of gravity and ensure comfort.
- Prioritize gentle stretches and movements that promote relaxation.

Guiding Principles for Adaptation:

a. Listen to Your Body:
- Pay attention to how your body responds during and after each session.
- If any movement causes discomfort, adapt or skip it to prioritize your well-being.

b. Communicate with Instructors:
- In group settings or virtual classes, communicate any health concerns with instructors.
- Instructors can provide personalized guidance and modifications based on your needs.

c. Gradual Progression:
- Begin with foundational exercises and gradually progress as your fitness level improves.
- Avoid pushing beyond your comfort zone and prioritize consistency over intensity.

d. Individualized Modifications:
- Work with your healthcare provider or a certified Pilates instructor to develop personalized modifications.
- Modifications may include variations in range of motion, props, or specific exercises tailored to your condition.

Chapter 3
The Complete Wall Pilates Routine
Full Body Wall Pilates Workout

Welcome to the heart of your Wall Pilates journey! This chapter unveils the comprehensive Full Body Wall Pilates Workout, a harmonious blend of exercises designed to invigorate your entire being. As we delve into the routine, each movement becomes a brushstroke, contributing to the masterpiece of your physical and mental well-being. Let's embark on this transformative journey, step by step, with detailed illustrations to guide you through the graceful motions.

In this section, we present a carefully crafted Full Body Wall Pilates Workout, uniting various poses to target every muscle group. This routine is designed to enhance strength, flexibility, and balance, offering a holistic approach to your fitness journey.

Before You Begin: Warm-Up
- Start with gentle stretches and warm-up exercises to prepare your body for the upcoming routine.
- Incorporate breathing techniques to center your mind and connect with your breath.
- Ensure your Wall Pilates space is set up with proper equipment and a supportive wall.

Full Body Wall Pilates Workout: Step-by-Step Guide

a. The Wall Lean (2 minutes):

- Stand facing the wall with feet hip-width apart.
- Place your palms against the wall at shoulder height.
- Lean forward, maintaining a straight line from head to heels.
- Engage your core and hold the position for 30 seconds.
- Repeat for a total of 2 minutes.

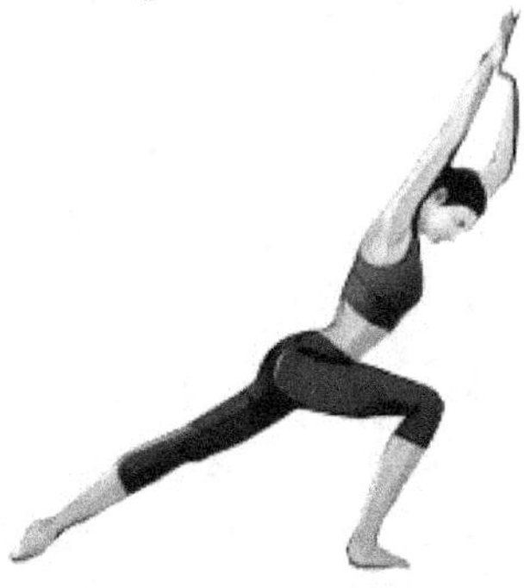

b. Wall Squats (3 sets of 12 repetitions):

- Position your back against the wall with feet shoulder-width apart.
- Lower into a seated position, as if sitting in an imaginary chair.
- Ensure knees are directly above ankles.
- Perform 12 repetitions for each set, gradually increasing as you progress.

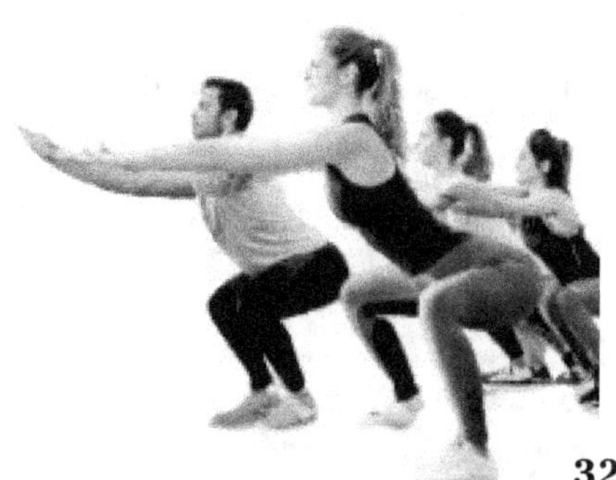

- Face the wall and place your hands on it at shoulder height.
- Step back until your body is in a straight line from head to heels.
- Engage your core and hold the plank position for 30 seconds.
- Rest for 15 seconds between sets.

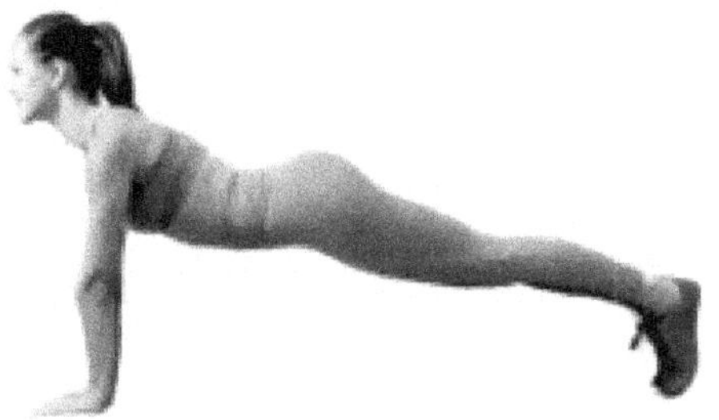

d. Wall Bridge (3 sets of 15 repetitions):

- Lie on your back with feet flat against the wall and knees bent.
- Press your lower back into the floor, engaging your core.
- Lift your hips toward the ceiling, creating a straight line from shoulders to knees.
- Lower your hips back down with control.
- Perform 15 repetitions for each set.

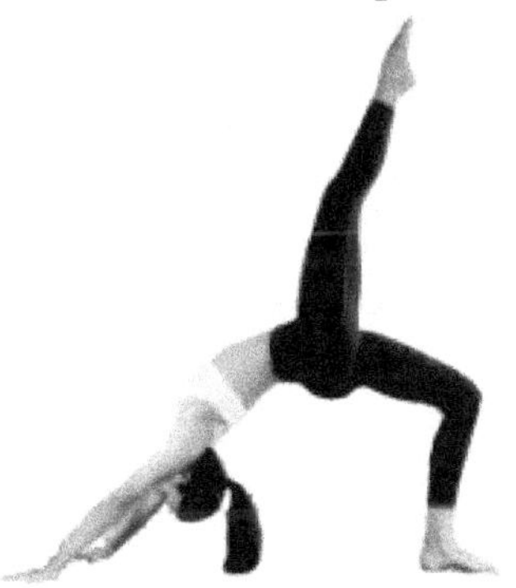

e. Wall Leg Lifts (2 sets of 10 repetitions each leg):

- Stand facing the wall, placing your hands on it for support.
- Lift one leg straight back, engaging your glutes.
- Lower the leg back down with control.
- Repeat for 10 repetitions on each leg.

f. Wall Roll Down (2 sets of 8 repetitions):

- Stand with your back against the wall and feet hip-width apart.
- Slowly roll down, articulating through your spine.
- Roll back up to the starting position with control.
- Repeat for 8 repetitions.

Adapting the Routine to Your Pace: A Personalized Approach to Wall Pilates

In the dynamic journey of Wall Pilates, the key to a sustainable and enjoyable practice lies in adapting the routine to your unique pace. This chapter is dedicated to empowering you with the freedom to personalize your Wall Pilates experience, ensuring that it aligns seamlessly with your fitness level, goals, and comfort. Let's explore the art of adapting the routine to your pace, making each movement a mindful and empowering expression of your wellness journey.

Understanding Your Individual Pace:
Before delving into the adaptations, it's crucial to recognize the value of understanding your individual pace. Your pace is a combination of your fitness level, comfort with specific movements, and the rhythm that feels most natural to you. It's not a race; it's a personalized journey where every step, stretch, and breath is guided by your unique needs.

Adapting the Full Body Wall Pilates Routine:

a. Duration of Poses:

Standard Pace:
- Follow the recommended duration for each pose in the routine.
- This pace is suitable for those comfortable with the outlined timings.

Adaptation:
- If you prefer a slower pace, extend the duration of each pose.
- If you prefer a faster pace, shorten the duration while maintaining proper form.

b. Number of Repetitions:

Standard Pace:
- Perform the suggested number of repetitions for each exercise in the routine.
- This pace provides a balanced challenge for various fitness levels.

Adaptation:
- If you prefer a gentler approach, reduce the number of repetitions.
- If you're seeking a more intense workout, increase the repetitions gradually.

c. Transition Time Between Poses:

Standard Pace:
- Allow a brief rest or transition time between each pose, as outlined in the routine.
- This pace supports a steady flow and focused performance.

Adaptation:
- If you desire a more meditative experience, extend the transition time.
- If you prefer a more energetic flow, minimize the rest periods between poses.

Standard Pace:
- Follow the structured rest intervals suggested in the routine.
- This pace balances exertion and recovery for an efficient workout.

Adaptation:
- If you need more rest, take additional breaks as needed.
- If you prefer continuous movement, reduce the rest intervals while staying mindful of your body's signals.

Listening to Your Body:
The most crucial aspect of adapting the routine to your pace is cultivating a deep connection with your body. Listen to its cues, honor its limitations, and celebrate its strengths. If a certain pose feels challenging, modify it to suit your comfort level. If you're yearning for a bit more intensity, explore gradual progressions that align with your capabilities.

Guiding Principles for Personalization:

a. Consistency Over Intensity:
- Prioritize consistency in your practice rather than pushing for intense workouts.
- Gradually increase intensity as your body becomes accustomed to the routine.

b. Mindful Movement:

- Embrace mindful movement, paying attention to how each pose feels.
- Adjust your pace based on your breath, ensuring a harmonious flow.

c. Progress at Your Own Rate:

- Your fitness journey is unique, and progress varies for each individual.
- Celebrate small victories and progress at a rate that feels comfortable and sustainable.

d. Seek Professional Guidance:

- If you're unsure about adaptations, consider seeking guidance from a certified Pilates instructor.
- Instructors can provide personalized recommendations based on your goals and fitness level.

Embrace Your Pace, Celebrate Your Progress:

As you navigate the Full Body Wall Pilates Routine, let the rhythm be your own. Whether you choose to move gracefully through each pose or savor moments of stillness, remember that the beauty of Wall Pilates lies in its adaptability. Your pace is an integral part of your wellness journey, and as you adapt the routine to suit your needs, each movement becomes a celebration of your unique strength and dedication. Embrace your pace, honor your body, and revel in the transformative power of Wall Pilates personalized just for you.

b. Mindful Movement:

- Embrace mindful movement, paying attention to how each pose feels.
- Adjust your pace based on your breath, ensuring a harmonious flow.

c. Progress at Your Own Rate:

- Your fitness journey is unique, and progress varies for each individual.
- Celebrate small victories and progress at a rate that feels comfortable and sustainable.

d. Seek Professional Guidance:

- If you're unsure about adaptations, consider seeking guidance from a certified Pilates instructor.
- Instructors can provide personalized recommendations based on your goals and fitness level.

Embrace Your Pace, Celebrate Your Progress:
As you navigate the Full Body Wall Pilates Routine, let the rhythm be your own. Whether you choose to move gracefully through each pose or savor moments of stillness, remember that the beauty of Wall Pilates lies in its adaptability. Your pace is an integral part of your wellness journey, and as you adapt the routine to suit your needs, each movement becomes a celebration of your unique strength and dedication. Embrace your pace, honor your body, and revel in the transformative power of Wall Pilates personalized just for you.

Targeted Exercises for Specific Benefits

In the realm of Wall Pilates, the art of targeted exercises takes center stage, offering a tailored approach to meet specific fitness goals. This chapter unveils a curated selection of exercises designed to hone in on distinct benefits – from building strength and enhancing flexibility to refining balance.

1. Building Strength: The Pillars of Power

a. Wall Squats:

Execution:

- Stand with your back against the wall and feet shoulder-width apart.
- Lower into a seated position, keeping knees directly above ankles.
- Engage core muscles and push through heels to return to the starting position.

Benefits:

- Targets quadriceps, hamstrings, and glutes for lower body strength.
- Engages core muscles, contributing to overall abdominal strength.

Execution:
- Face the wall, place palms on it at shoulder height, arms extended.
- Lower your chest toward the wall by bending elbows.
- Push back to the starting position.

Benefits:
- Strengthens chest, shoulders, triceps, and core.
- Provides a modified push-up option for varying fitness levels.

c. Wall Plank:

Execution:
- Face the wall, place hands on it at shoulder height.
- Step back until body forms a straight line from head to heels.
- Engage core and hold the plank position.

Benefits:
- Activates core, shoulders, and arms for overall upper body strength.
- Enhances stability and endurance.

2. Enhancing Flexibility: The Flow of Fluidity

a. Wall Forward Fold:

Execution:
- Stand facing the wall with feet hip-width apart.
- Place palms on the wall at shoulder height and hinge at the hips.
- Allow the upper body to fold forward, feeling a gentle stretch.

Benefits:
- Stretches hamstrings, lower back, and shoulders.
- Promotes flexibility in the spine and improves overall body mobility.

b. Wall Chest Opener:

Execution:
- Stand with your side to the wall, arm extended and palm placed on it.
- Gently rotate your torso away from the wall, opening the chest.
- Feel a stretch across the chest and shoulders.

Benefits:
- Releases tension in chest and shoulders, enhancing upper body flexibility.
- Improves range of motion in the torso.

Execution:
- Sit close to the wall with one leg extended up, foot flexed.
- Reach toward your toes, feeling a stretch along the back of the extended leg.

Benefits:
- Stretches hamstrings and calves, promoting lower body flexibility.
- Enhances flexibility in the hip flexors.

3. Improving Balance: The Poise of Precision

Execution:
- Stand facing the wall with feet hip-width apart.
- Lift one foot off the ground, bringing the knee toward your chest.
- Hold the position, balancing on one leg.

Benefits:
- Enhances stability and proprioception.
- Strengthens ankle and lower leg muscles, improving overall balance.

b. Wall Tree Pose:

Execution:
- Stand with your side to the wall, placing one foot on the inner thigh of the opposite leg.
- Bring hands to heart center and balance.
- Use the wall for support as needed.

Benefits:
- Improves balance and concentration.
- Strengthens muscles in the standing leg and engages core stability.

c. Wall Plank with Leg Lift:

Execution:
- Face the wall in a plank position.
- Lift one leg off the ground, keeping it straight.
- Hold briefly, then switch legs.

Benefits:
- Challenges stability and balance in a dynamic plank variation.
- Strengthens core, shoulders, and legs.

Guiding Principles for Targeted Exercises:

a. Consistency is Key:
- Incorporate targeted exercises consistently to experience meaningful benefits.
- Gradually progress by increasing repetitions or holding positions for longer durations.

b. Listen to Your Body:

- Adapt exercises based on your comfort level and any existing physical considerations.
- If an exercise feels challenging, modify it to ensure proper form and safety.

c. Variety Enhances Results:

- Integrate a variety of targeted exercises into your routine for a well-rounded approach.
- Each exercise contributes uniquely to your strength, flexibility, and balance.

d. Personalize Your Routine:

- Tailor your routine by selecting exercises that align with your specific fitness goals.
- Experiment with different combinations to keep your routine engaging and effective.

In the symphony of targeted exercises, each movement contributes to the harmony of your overall well-being. Whether you seek to build strength, enhance flexibility, or improve balance, the wall becomes a versatile ally in your fitness journey. Embrace the precision of each exercise, savor the fluidity of movement, and revel in the poise of balance. Let targeted exercises be the cornerstone of your Wall Pilates practice, sculpting a body that is strong, flexible, and gracefully balanced.

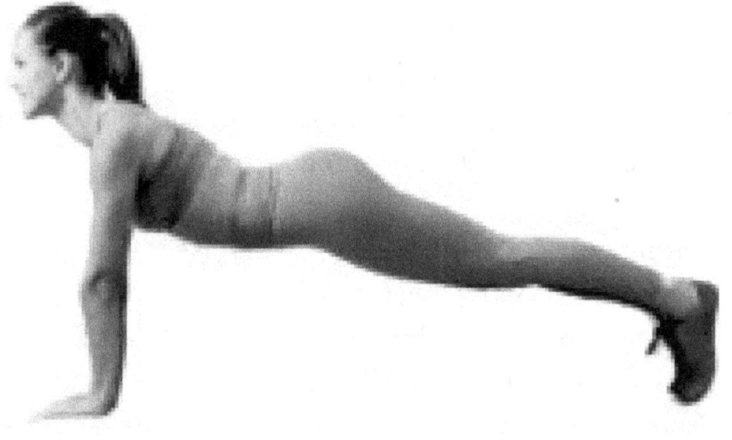

Chapter 4
Integrating Wall Pilates into Daily Life
Incorporating Short Workouts into Your Day

In the fast-paced rhythm of modern life, finding time for exercise can be a challenge. This chapter is dedicated to unraveling the secret of integrating short yet effective workouts into your busy day. Discover the art of seizing moments for movement, transforming your daily schedule into an opportunity for wellness.

1. The Power of Short Workouts:

Short workouts, often referred to as micro-workouts, are potent bursts of activity designed to maximize efficiency and impact. While they may be brief, their benefits extend far beyond their duration. Here's why incorporating short workouts into your day is a game-changer:

a. Accessibility:

- Short workouts require minimal time and space, making them accessible to anyone, anywhere.
- You can perform them at home, in the office, or even during a break in your daily routine.

b. Consistency is Achievable:

- Short workouts are easier to integrate into a busy schedule, fostering consistency.
- The regularity of brief sessions contributes to cumulative health benefits over time.

c. Mental Refreshment:
- A quick workout serves as a mental break, rejuvenating your focus and energy.
- Physical activity has been shown to enhance cognitive function and reduce stress.

d. Tailored to Busy Lifestyles:
- Short workouts cater to the demands of modern lifestyles, accommodating tight schedules.
- They eliminate the common barrier of time constraints, allowing everyone to prioritize fitness.

2. Quick Sessions for Busy Schedules:

Now, let's explore a set of quick sessions that seamlessly integrate into your day, requiring minimal time commitment.

a. Morning Energizer (5 minutes):

Routine:
- Jumping jacks: 1 minute
- Bodyweight squats: 1 minute
- Wall push-ups: 1 minute
- High knees: 1 minute
- Plank: 1 minute

Benefits:
- Boosts morning energy levels.
- Engages major muscle groups.
- Sets a positive tone for the day.

b. Lunch Break Revitalizer (7 minutes):

Routine:
- Wall sit: 1 minute
- Standing leg raises: 1 minute each leg
- Desk push-ups: 1 minute
- Forward folds: 1 minute
- Seated twists: 1 minute each side
- Standing calf raises: 1 minute

Benefits:
- Counteracts midday fatigue.
- Promotes circulation and flexibility.
- Enhances mental clarity.

c. Post-Work Pick-Me-Up (10 minutes):

Routine:
- Quick jog in place: 2 minutes
- Lunges: 2 minutes
- Tricep dips using a sturdy surface: 2 minutes
- Mountain climbers: 2 minutes
- Wall plank: 2 minutes

Benefits:
- Releases endorphins after work.
- Targets cardiovascular fitness and strength.
- Provides a healthy transition from work to personal time.

3. Strategies for Successful Integration:

a. Schedule with Intent:

- Block out specific times for short workouts in your daily schedule.
- Treat these sessions with the same importance as other appointments.

b. Make it a Habit:

c. Mental Refreshment:

- A quick workout serves as a mental break, rejuvenating your focus and energy.
- Physical activity has been shown to enhance cognitive function and reduce stress.

d. Tailored to Busy Lifestyles:

- Short workouts cater to the demands of modern lifestyles, accommodating tight schedules.
- They eliminate the common barrier of time constraints, allowing everyone to prioritize fitness.

2. Quick Sessions for Busy Schedules:

Now, let's explore a set of quick sessions that seamlessly integrate into your day, requiring minimal time commitment.

a. Morning Energizer (5 minutes):

Routine:

- Jumping jacks: 1 minute
- Bodyweight squats: 1 minute
- Wall push-ups: 1 minute
- High knees: 1 minute
- Plank: 1 minute

Benefits:
- Boosts morning energy levels.
- Engages major muscle groups.
- Sets a positive tone for the day.

b. Lunch Break Revitalizer (7 minutes):

Routine:
- Wall sit: 1 minute
- Standing leg raises: 1 minute each leg
- Desk push-ups: 1 minute
- Forward folds: 1 minute
- Seated twists: 1 minute each side
- Standing calf raises: 1 minute

Benefits:
- Counteracts midday fatigue.
- Promotes circulation and flexibility.
- Enhances mental clarity.

c. Post-Work Pick-Me-Up (10 minutes):

Routine:
- Quick jog in place: 2 minutes
- Lunges: 2 minutes
- Tricep dips using a sturdy surface: 2 minutes
- Mountain climbers: 2 minutes
- Wall plank: 2 minutes

Benefits:
- Releases endorphins after work.
- Targets cardiovascular fitness and strength.

- Provides a healthy transition from work to personal time.

3. Strategies for Successful Integration:

a. Schedule with Intent:
- Block out specific times for short workouts in your daily schedule.
- Treat these sessions with the same importance as other appointments.

b. Make it a Habit:
- Consistency is key. Establish a routine by consistently incorporating short workouts at the same times each day.
- Turn your micro-workouts into a habitual part of your daily life.

c. Break it Up:
- If time permits, break your short workouts into even smaller segments throughout the day.
- Consider a few minutes in the morning, during lunch, and in the evening.

d. Embrace Variety:
- Keep things interesting by varying your exercises.
- Explore different routines to target various muscle groups and maintain engagement.

Conclusion

As we conclude this transformative exploration into the realm of "Wall Pilates for Seniors Over 60," the pages of this guide are not merely the conclusion of a book; they mark the commencement of a flourishing journey towards holistic well-being. Through the lens of controlled movements against the wall, mindful breaths, and intentional exercises, we've uncovered a tapestry of benefits that extend far beyond physical fitness.

From the tangible improvements in strength, flexibility, and balance to the subtle yet profound impact on mental clarity and emotional resilience, Wall Pilates emerges as a catalyst for positive change. This isn't just a guide to exercises; it's an invitation to cultivate a life imbued with vitality, clarity, and a deep connection to oneself.

In the quiet moments of mindful movement, you've discovered not only the strength of your muscles but also the resilience of your spirit. The intentional breaths have not only fueled your physical endeavors but have become whispers of tranquility, dissipating the stresses of the day. As you've delved into the poses against the wall, you've uncovered not just a workout routine but a sanctuary where physical, mental, and emotional well-being converge.

This guide is a testament to the idea that age is not a limitation but a canvas upon which we can paint a vibrant tapestry of our well-lived lives. It's a celebration of the wisdom that comes with each intentional movement, the joy that arises from the harmony of mind and body, and the fulfillment found in the pursuit of a balanced and meaningful life.

As you close these pages, remember that the mat against the wall is not just a physical space; it's a haven for transformation. Your journey with Wall Pilates is an ongoing narrative, where each breath, each stretch, and each moment of mindful engagement contributes to the unfolding story of your well-being.

May the principles you've embraced within these chapters accompany you beyond the mat, enriching every facet of your life. May your days be filled with the energy derived from strength, the clarity found in mindful moments, and the resilience that comes from intentional living.

Let this conclusion be the prologue to a chapter of your life where well-being is not just a destination but a continuous journey one that unfolds with grace, purpose, and an ever-growing sense of vitality. The mat against the wall is your canvas; paint it with the colors of joy, balance, and fulfillment. Here's to the flourishing journey that lies ahead.